# DETOXIFICATION
## A SENSIBLE METHOD FOR MAINTAINING OPTIMIM HEALTH

D1036315

**Ruth Sackman**

**Foundation for Advancement in Cancer Therapy**

DETOXIFICATION-A SENSIBLE METHOD
FOR MAINTAINING OPTIMUM HEALTH

Foundation for Advancement in Cancer Therapy (F.A.C.T.)
P.O. Box 1242
Old Chelsea Station
New York, NY 10113

Typography by Alliance Printing
Cover Art Paper Sculpture by Ellen Rixford Studios
Printed in the United States of America

ISBN: 978-0-9702061-0-7

# TABLE OF CONTENTS

*Dedicated to my son*
*Howard Sackman and*
*my grandchildren*
*Lisa and Bart*

# PREFACE

After 35 years of experience as president of the Foundation for Advancement in Cancer Therapy, (FACT), guiding cancer patients to achieve better host resistance to overcome cancer or, to avoid a recurrence of cancer, it became evident that what could cure cancer or avoid a recurrence, would be capable of preventing cancer and other degenerative health conditions. Preventing cancer or other chronic health problems makes more sense than being careless and facing the ordeal and emotional turmoil of curing the disease.

Chemical pollutants in the air we breathe, the water we drink and the food we eat are certainly suspected contributors to producing cancer. Actually, some of the pesticides that have been approved are *actually known carcinogens*. Knowing how to avoid most of the hazards of a chemical buildup that can produce a dreaded disease such as cancer or other degenerative diseases and, if exposed, knowing how to alleviate the toxicity, should make disease preventable in most instances.

If cancer can be avoided, we can assume that the same concepts are capable of protecting us from other chronic diseases.

I

# INTRODUCTION

This book is about the buildup of toxicity from pesticides and other unnatural material added to our food, air and water that is causing a myriad of health problems which plague us and make our lives uncomfortable. It is about how we can control the toxic buildup and gain freedom from the discomfort of toxicity and achieve the restoration and maintenance of good health and the enjoyment of life.

We are a nation of people who are doctoring for all sorts of ailments. Our hospital complexes and doctors' offices are filled with patients. And the pharmaceutical companies are probably the richest in the world. Someone might say, "But it must be all right, life expectancy is going up." True. But is it because adding chemicals to our food, air and water are making people healthier and extending life expectancy? I don't think so. I believe it is because surgical procedures are much more skillful and adding years to a person's life. I think some of the additional time is due to the expertise of doctors' skill in microsurgery, heart, liver and kidney transplants, heart bypasses and other skillful techniques. Or, could keeping people alive artificially on life-support systems be raising the average?

I also believe the improvement in life expectancy is due to the health movement which has grown to a twenty-two billion dollar industry. People have become more active in preventive health than they were years ago. As a matter of fact, people interested in nutrition not more than thirty years ago earned the label "health nut." Today many of those same critics are seeking the very same information for themselves and following healthier, preventive lifestyles. It is interesting to note that, in spite of all the money spent on health care in the United States, we are about 26th on the life expectancy list.

From my long years of experience helping cancer patients, I believe that we can avoid many of the health problems that plague us, including cancer. And we can correct most of them if we understand how our bodies develop complications, the causes of a biochemical breakdown and how we store toxins from our polluted lifestyle and environment and the impact of those toxins on our health. We can learn how to minimize the toxic buildup and how to eliminate the toxic accumulation from our bodies.

We live in a polluted world: Chemicals are added to our food to avoid salmonella, to add shelf life, to make the food look more appealing, and numerous other reasons as though the chemicals are absolutely safe. We frequently take medicine to alleviate minor uncomfortable symptoms. Chemicals are poured into our drinking water for purification, trees are sprayed with insect repellents and we breathe in the fumes. Since it seems impossible to avoid completely the poisons in our food, water, air and environment, we need a method to eliminate the toxins periodically so that they do not accumulate to the point of causing health problems which require treatment or might be irreparable.

I will try to spell out the complications with which we live, the way our bodies handle the toxic elements and how we can get relief with detoxification. With better understanding of how we develop chronic degenerative diseases for which we are constantly medicating, we might be able to avoid the pitfalls. By addressing the causes which can, and usually do, stem from an accumulation of toxic substances from our polluted food, air and water, we especially might be able to avoid the chronic degenerative diseases which tend to make life unbearable,

There are a number of ways in which we can detoxify our bodies. One chapter will describe some of them so we can choose the one with which we are most comfortable and, the one most suitable for our lifestyle. If there is any doubt about making a choice, I suggest that it be discussed with a doctor or other professional resource.

Eliminating toxicity will clear the mind, relax the nerves and add zest to our life.

# Acknowledgements

This book could not have been written if it were not for the valuable and extensive knowledge I gained from the most qualified practitioners in the field of natural healing. These men and women pioneered the concepts which are the guidelines for the health movement today. Many of them developed their skill through hard work and an innate sense of what was logical and a high regard for the Hippocratic concept—"first do no harm."

I had the good fortune to establish a mutually respectful relationship with these outstanding men and women and they were generous in providing me with their vast knowledge by guiding me to the right books, sending me publications from their extensive collections, having many discussions over dinner and the telephone, etc. I am so grateful that words cannot possibly express the depth of my gratitude.

I hesitate listing their names for fear of omitting someone but they need to be recognized.
They are:
* Dr. Karl Aly, M.D, Director of a 90 bed clinic in Sweden which uses the Waerland Health System.
* Dr. Jesse Mercer Gehman, D.C. was the President of an international organization of Natural Practitioners. We had many health discussions over the telephone late in the evening. He then followed up by sharing material from his vast library of printed material.

* Dr. Karl O. Heede, M.D., a specialist in the Waerland Health System. .

* Dr. Bernard Jensen was the Director of the Hidden Valley Health Ranch in Escondido, California. Dr. Jensen, was a world renowned iridologist and author of numerous health books.

* Dr. William D. Kelley, D.D.S., was the creator of a Metabolic Health System and author of the book, *One Answer to Cancer.* .

* Dr. Alan Nittler, M.D. had a nutritional practice in northern California and was the author of the book, *New Breed of Doctor.*

* Dr. Leo Roy, M.D. spent 6 months working with Dr. Max Gerson at his health clinic in Nanuet, New York and travelled to clinics worldwide to hone his extensive knowledge. Dr. Max Gerson was the author of the book, *A Cancer Therapy, Results of Fifty Cases.*

* Ebba Waerland worked with her husband, Are Waerland, at the original Waerland Clinic in Sweden and authored the book, *Rebuilding Health.*

*Dr. Norman Walker was the author of many health books and the developer of the vegetable juice extractor. I was fortunate to be able to talk to him on the telephone a few times but his books were the best source of knowledge about health.

* Dr. Max Warmbrand, a Naturopath who had a practice in Connecticut for about sixty years, was also the author of numerous health books which, sadly, are now out of print.

. .      So many of these masters of healing are no longer

available for this generation to glean their precious knowledge directly from them.

I also want to thank all the people who graciously volunteered to help me with this booklet: Consuelo Reyes, Josephine Coppa, Ellen Rixford and Corinne Loreto, They helped with the format, editing, typing and valuable suggestions. All of which were so helpful in knowing whether the material was written in clear language so that it would be understood by the readers.

# Chapter 1

# Sources of Toxicity

*At least 85% of all cancer is caused by man-made products*
*— Irving Selikoff, M.D.*

We live in the chemical age. We are bombarded with toxins from unexpected and unbelievable sources. The food we eat, the water we drink and the air we breathe are loaded with toxic chemicals, and the drugs used today are primarily chemical. All of this may be beyond what the human system can tolerate and still maintain good health unless we try to control the toxic buildup, and periodically take steps to eliminate it.

## FOOD

Let's start with the food supply as this is the fuel that repairs organs and generates the energy that makes our bodies function, just as gasoline makes a car go. Chemicals added to food are used from the seed to the table. The seeds are coated with chemicals or genetically engineered (GE) with added pesticides so that the farmer can avoid the need for some of the pesticide spraying, nevertheless, he still sprays to avoid having the crop destroyed by insects. Much of our food is processed by canning, freezing or irradiation

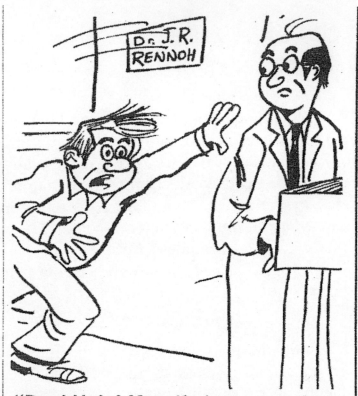

"Doc! Help! My wife just served me potassium sorbate, mono and di-glycerites, guar gum, cocoa pro-cessed with alkalai, carrageenan and polysorbate 80!!"

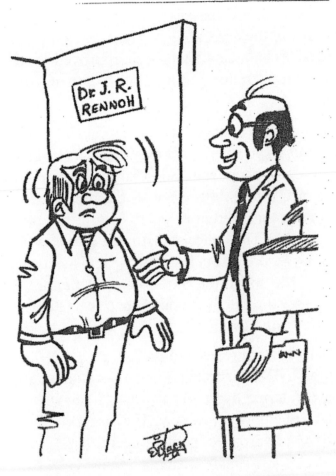

"Oh, you mean Ice cream?"

to which food processors add chemical preservatives, stabilizers, coloring for cosmetic purposes, sweeteners, flavor enhancers and whatever is approved by the Food and Drug Administration (FDA) that they think is necessary to deliver their product to the consumer safely, attractively and tasty. About 30,000 chemicals have been approved by the Food and Drug Administration (FDA). Not all of them *guaranteed to be safe.*

Following is a lunch menu compiled by a health publication about 15 years ago that may give you an insight into the typical use of chemicals. Some of the chemicals may no longer be in use possibly because the dangerous level of toxicity was recognized after years of use, but others may have been added. The concept is still the same. A few of the items may be nontoxic, but most are toxic. I am sure that you will not want to spend the time to read the entire list but I want you to see the extent of added chemicals that you might ingest *in just one meal.*

**Juice:** Benzoic Acid (preservative)
Dimethyil polysiloxane (anti-foaming agent).
**Fruit cup:** Calcium hypochlorite (germicide wash)
Sodium chloride (prevents browning)
Sodium hydroxide (peeling agent)
Calcium hydroxide (firming agent)
Sodium metasilicate (peeling for peaches)
Sorbic acid (fungistat)
Sulfur dioxide (preservative)
FD&C red #3 (coloring for maraschino cherries)

**Soup:** Butylated hydroxyanisole (antioxidant)
Sodium phosphate dibasic (emulsion for tomato soup
Citric acid (dispersant in soup base)

**Sandwich with meat processed and cheese:**
Sodium diacetate (mold inhibitor)
Mono-diglyceride (emulsifier)
Potassium bromate (maturing agent)
Aluminum phosphate (improver)
Calcium phosphate monobasic (dough conditioner)
Chloramine T (flour bleach)
Aluminum potassium sulfate (baking powder ingredient)
Sodium or potassium nitrate (color fixative)
Sodium chloride (preservative)
Guar gum (binder)
Hydrogen peroxide (bleach)
FD&C Yellow #3 (coloring)
Nordihydroguairetic acid (antioxidant)
Alkanate (dye)
Methylviolet (marking ink)
Asafoetidc (onion flavoring)
Sodium phosphate (buffer)
Magnesium carbonate (drying agent)
Calcium propionate (preservative)
Calcium citrate (plasticiser)
Sodium citrate (emulsifier)
Sodium alginate (stabilizer)
Pyroligneous acid (smoke flavor)

**Ice cream:** Amylacetate (banana flavoring)
Vanilidine kectone (imitation vanilla flavoring)

# WATER

*"It has become obvious that man today has the awesome genius to completely poison every living thing on the face of the earth and in the waters below. Most of this has come about through man's efforts to make life easier — mitigating pain and disease, bringing the world closer to his living room through communication, pursuing his quest into outer space and making destructive elements of war.*

*"Most of this is caused by man's creation of new but deadly chemical compounds."*

(The above item appeared in the Natural Food Associates (NFA) official publication. NFA is a nonprofit organization concerned about the proliferation of chemicals in farming as well as water and food.)

Toxins in the water come from numerous sources. Bacteriacides are added to control germs. Pesticides are sprayed on lawns, trees and crops. When it rains the water runs off into the rivers, lakes and ponds carrying the chemical soup. In some instances, factories dump their waste into the rivers, streams and on the earth which usually seeps down into the rivers (aquifers) below ground. These underground rivers provide water for populations that rely on springs and wells.

The clouds collect chemicals from smoke stacks that spew fumes into the air that ultimately come down to earth as acid rain. In many cities and towns, fluoride is deliberately added to drinking water. Fluoride is a toxic waste product of the aluminum industry, agribusiness and glass manufacturing. Although fluoride is a poison, some people have been convinced that it will cut down on tooth decay. Unfortunately, that concept does not consider the damage it is doing to the person's body. It affects metabolism, cuts down on the body's use of calcium and causes mottled teeth. One study claims it causes cancer, and probably other complications. A cancer study done by Dr. John Yiamouyiannis, a biochemist, showed a 10% rise in cancer in fluoridated cities compared to unfluoridated comparable cities. It would be in the interest of society if some method other than adding fluoride to our precious *drinking water* would be used by the companies who need to dispose of this waste product.

## AIR

Toxins in the air come from factories such as the oil refining industry, factories that use coal or oil, especially coal in the manufacturing process, exhaust fumes from cars, trucks, planes and construction equipment, etc. Many cities burn their trash which adds to the air pollution. Household cleaners give off fumes that we breathe in while tidying up our homes. Some of the elements polluting our air are benzene, polyvinyl chloride, vinyl chloride, asbestos, nitrosomines, etc. No doubt there are numerous other instances that contribute to air pollution. A recent study reported: When pregnant mothers were exposed to air pollution, there was an affect on the genes of their offspring.

## DRUGS

Medicine today is mostly chemical and, when prescribed, is usually taken daily and more than once a day. Many pills are coated with coloring. Capsules are another source of coloring. Binders, preservatives and other unpronounceable elements are used in the manufacturing process. Drugs are often approved that are so toxic that after being out in the marketplace and used by *millions of patients,* the dangers that did not show up during research become obvious and the drugs are withdrawn. Some pharmaceuticals have caused death, suicidal tendency, heart failure and other serious health hazards. This is a logical and urgent reason for us to detoxify periodically.

Following is a list of drugs, compiled in the year 2000 by the Consumer Healthcare Products Association (CHPA) that were considered toxic because they contained phenylpropanolamine (PPA). The study was done at Yale University. It was supported financially by CHPA which then disavowed the study because it was not in their financial interest, although it was important for the consumer's health. FDA then recommended (not mandated) that the drugs containing PPA be removed from the marketplace. As usual, the trade groups disagreed and said they would consider the recommendation. Many of the items were over-the-counter and readily available to the consumer. I am listing them so you can see the extent of the problem.

Acutrim,

      Alka-Seltzer Plus Children's Cold Medicine
      BC Allergy Sinus Cold Powder
      BC Sinus Cold Powder
      Comtrex Deep Chest Cold & Congestion Relief
      Comtrex Flu Therapy & Fever Relief Day & Night
      Contac 12 Hour Cold Capsules
      Contac 12 Hour Cold Caplets

Cold, Flu & Sinus

      Dexatrim Caffeine Free
      Dexatrim Extended Duration\ Dexatrim Gelcaps
      Dexatrim Vitamin C/Caffeine Free
      Dimetapp Cold & Allergy Chewable Tablets
      Dimetapp Cold & Cough Liquid
      Dimetapp DM Cold & Cough Elixir
      Naldecon DX Pediatric Drops
      Robitussin CF
      Triaminic DM Cough Relief
      Triaminic Syrup Cold & Allergy

## COSMETICS

Until recently, the FDA did very little about checking on the safety of cosmetics. In February 2005 the agency sent a strongly worded message to the Cosmetics, Toiletry and Fragrance Industry (a trade group that represents 600 manufacturers) that they will evaluate cosmetic safety more energetically in 2005. This is being done at the urging of a group of toxicologists, biologists, environmentalists and people in the public health field.

A list of 100 ingredients used in cosmetics included formaldehyde (thought to produce cancer). Twenty-four of the 100 items were suspected of causing birth defects and 20 others were considered capable of harming the nervous system.

Coloring agents in hair dyes are known to be absorbed through the skin and ultimately found in body fluids.

Cosmetics are rarely considered as containing harmful substances, so exercising a little caution by reading labels may be in your interest.

## GENETIC MODIFICATION (GM)

This is a fairly recent phenomenon. (Seeds are altered by combining them genetically with pesticides to ward off insects or other alien elements. Modifications in the genetic components are often designed to maintain shelf-life for a longer time or just for cosmetic purposes). Research as to the safety is questionable. Twenty or so years from now, it may become known that not only were GM foods harmful to insects, but to humans as well and possibly caused irreparable harm. Unfortunately, that happens much too frequently for us to be complacent about so-called "scientific research" that claims an additive or a process is absolutely safe. The research for safety usually is done on mice which is not comparable to the human system.

With this barrage of material, it is easily understood

why we need to add detoxification to our lifestyle. Nature has a built-in system (the immune system) to help the body detoxify which is probably why we don't die immediately from ingesting toxic substances. But the amount of toxins that we absorb daily usually goes far beyond the body's normal capacity to eliminate all of the poison. If the body's immune system is too overloaded and cannot eliminate all the poison, the remainder is then stored in the tissue, fat and lymphatic system. This can build up for years and then manifest in a chronic degenerative health problem and not be recognized as toxicity.

## ENZYMATIC FUNCTION

Toxins undermine competent enzymatic function; a *very serious health hazard*. Weak enzymatic function interferes with the body's ability to metabolize (digest) its food properly. Since enzymatic function is linked to the liver, pancreas and endocrine system (thyroid, adrenals, pituitary, etc.), a weakness in any of the organs of the endocrine system will interfere with competent metabolism. This undigested food becomes a waste product that the body seeks ways to discard. If it cannot because of overloading of the elimination system, the waste will be added to the buildup of toxins in storage. Poor enzymatic function is a catalyst for developing health complications.

One consequence of inadequate metabolism, of course, would be production of deficient cells. Could this be a cause of cancer?

# .STRESS

This is the most disregarded complication in maintaining an efficiently functioning body. The mind is actually in control of the well-being of the body to achieve healing or in maintaining health. ***Stress plays havoc with all body functions,*** especially and including the endocrine system. The heart beats erratically affecting circulation, The bowel tenses, very often causing constipation or diarrhea. Breathing is irregular limiting oxygen intake. Digestion is compromised—a truly hazardous condition in our effort to regain and maintain health and produce healthy cells. The lymphatic system gets sluggish, slowing down natural detoxification, the immune system is compromised and nerve signals instructing the body's normal activity are skewed.

When the body is under stress and the food is not metabolized competently, ergo, becoming waste, and simultaneously, elimination is incomplete, the buildup of toxicity will be magnified putting the body in a vulnerable condition to develop a chronic, degenerative health problem.

# Chapter 2

# Health Problems that Develop from Toxicity

*We cannot afford to treat problems which arise from chemicals in foods as something distinct and uniquely different from those which arise from chemicals in drugs, air, soil or water. The human body doesn't differentiate between sources of environmental insults; it is the total impact on man that is the important concern.* —Dr. Alec B. Morrison, Deputy Director-General; of the Canadian Food and Drug Directorate.

## DIOXIN LINKED TO ILLS

Exposure to even small traces of dioxin, much of it through the food chain, poses wider health risks than had been suspected and may harm the human immune system and fetal development, a scientific study concluded. Dioxin is found in food packaging, paper towels, disposable diapers, and other products turned out by paper mills.

*Preliminary results of a study by Environmental Protection Agency (EPA) scientists suggests for the first time that cancer may not be the only troubling health concern posed by dioxin, a chlorine-based toxic compound present in the environment. Instead, the reassessment suggests, dioxin even at very common levels of exposure through the natural food chain may cause reproductive and de-*

*velopmental problems and suppress the human immune system. The scientists emphasized that the conclusions are based largely on animal studies.* — **Newsday, May 5, 1994** (note the time between this date and the date of the next item).

*On **June 12, 2000**, for the first time, the Environmental Protection Agency (EPA) declared that dioxin is a human carcinogen and said that a vast amount of exposure to the chemical comes from the food Americans eat. The EPA based the report on environmental health studies by ATSDR/CDC of human case studies involving a combination of epidemiological and mechanistic information, which indicate a causal relationship between exposure to dioxin and human cancer.* —from Day Cancer Research Foundation.

There was a six year gap between the first announcement and the second one before the EPA at least acknowledged seriously there was a problem with dioxin!

Despite scientific reports linking chemical pollutants to cancer and numerous other degenerative diseases, controversy always arises as the industry affected financially from negative research conclusions usually finances its own study, which usually claims that the information is inconclusive. This, understandably, causes confusion in the public mind. Unfortunately, human beings are the victims of these disagreements. That is why it is essential that individuals assume responsibility for their own safety and learn to recognize toxicity, know how to detoxify and *incorporate the procedure into their lifestyle.* It is possible for people to control the storage of toxins and maintain a body that does not store toxins until the degree of buildup causes an incurable degenerative disease.

## ENDOCRINE DISRUPTERS

A very serious complication with pesticide pollution is the fact that many pesticides mimic estrogen. These are called "endocrine disrupters."

Thus they are creating a hormonal imbalance causing an array of gynecological problems and male reproductive problems. *"Hormones are chemical messengers that travel in the bloodstream, turning on and off critical body functions to maintain health and well being. Hormones control growth, behavior in birds, fish, reptiles, amphibians and mammals, including humans,"* quoted from *Environment and Health Weekly.*

Animals have been born deformed, some with extra limbs. A frog was found with 2 heads, and numerous other strange deformities have appeared. If this happens to animals, can we conclude that it doesn't affect humans? Pesticides are creating a legacy of hormonal chaos.

Males are suffering from low sperm count and there is a suspicion that pollution affects the gender of humans. An article in *Science News* called these estrogen mimikers "Gender benders."

## THYROID FUNCTION

The pesticides that mimic estrogen creating a hormonal imbalance seem also to cause hypothyroidism (low thyroid function) which, in turn, can cause a mountain of health problems. One serious complication of hypothyroidism is inadequate calcium metabolism. Calcium is probably the most essential element in the food chain. It is needed to maintain the skeleton to avoid bone porosity, build blood, affect heart function and maintain healthy teeth and nails Since calcium is such an essential element in body function, Nature has provided it in nearly every vegetable, fruit, nut and grain. Inadequate thyroid function would deprive the body of its much-needed calcium metabolism leading to serious health complications, such as obesity, chronic fatigue, mental sluggishness, thinning hair, dry skin and a host of other problems.

## DRUGS

Many of the pesticides are known carcinogens. You may be surprized that the government agencies actually know this when they are approved. Approval is based on a yardstick that the FDA has established, but with which the consumer may not be completely comfortable. This yardstick is "benefit-risk-ratio" or "negligible risk." Although the FDA may feel comfortable with the risk, consumers may not be in agreement and therefore should investigate pestisides on their own.

Drug approval is based on the same benefit-risk concept. If you prefer to decide for yourself if *you* are willing to take the risk, it would be wise to look up the drugs, which your doctor prescribes, in the *Physicians Desk Reference (PDR\*)*, a book published for doctors which lists all drugs and their adverse reactions, dose, contraindications etc. The pharmaceutical industry prefers to list all of the hazards that it is aware of in order to help doctors make sound judgements for their patients and to avoid legal action because the patient was not informed. It will be obvious when you search the drug in the PDR that there are hazards in not considering the toxicity. You can then decide for yourself if you want to take the risk. There are many toxins in the food supply that we should try to guard against, but drugs are the *most* toxic and they are usually taken two or three times a day and taken over long-term. (The PDR\* can usually be found in medical libraries and in some public libraries.)

There are numerous drugs in the marketplace that have been approved by the Food and Drug Administration that *have not been proven safe*. The caveat by the pharmaceutical industry is to use as directed. Some of the drugs ultimately have to be withdrawn because they cause adverse health problems, including death. Many women took Hormone Replacement Therapy (HRT) because they were having uncomfortable symptoms of menopause, although it was known that HRT caused breast cancer. After years of use, by millions of people, it was also found to cause heart attacks and the consequence — death. Unfortunately, learning more about a drug after years of use is not unusual but common-place, as the FDA does not do the research but relies on the pharmaceutical industry to deliver the data for approval. Drug recalls are often made without much fanfare.

There was a 7% decrease in the incidence of breast cancer because many  women stopped taking HRT when the government publicly stated HRT was  causing serious heart problems. The diet pill Redux, the blood pressure drug Posicor and the pain killer Duract were recalled after years of use. Joe Graedon, a pharmacologist and Teresa Graedon, who has a doctorate in medical anthropology stated in an article in *Newsday*, "Redux affected the heart, Posicor showed an unexpected potential to interact in a deadly way with other medications and Duract prompted liver damage"

A report about Zoloft and Paxil, two of the mind-altering drugs commonly used to calm troubled people, including children, was found to cause suicidal tendencies. Hazardous discoveries, after years of use by patients, are not unusual but a common occurrence. Is it because it is not feasible for the research to be carried out for all the years required to reach these final conclusions?

It is interesting to note that as early as 1990  it was known that Paxil was dangerous. Not only was it *known then* to cause suicidal tendencies, but a Wyoming jury awarded $6.4 million dollars to the family of a man who killed two relatives and himself after taking the antidepressant. Paxil is only one of the mind-altering drugs in the marketplace. Anything that can distort a person's perspective, especially to that degree, must be toxic. Paxil is still available and still being prescribed by physicians.

Vioxx was withdrawn from the market in 2004 by the manufacturer  because it was causing heart problems. In

2005 a panel of scientists, doctors, etc., *selected by the FDA*, concluded that Vioxx could remain on the market if it was taken as directed). It was eventually withdrawn permanently. Another drug about which there has been negative reports is Fosamax, a drug widely used for osteoporosis. It is capable of damaging the esophagus, especially if swallowed without plenty of water.

## FRAGRANCES

Fragrances are rarely suspected of containing harmful chemicals .The following item has been excerpted from a study printed in the official publication of a group that is chemically sensitive. The study was of 13 harmful chemicals added to fragrances. I have elected to reprint the Benzyl Acetate item as I felt it was the most representative. It has been edited slightly to make it more understandable.

*BENZYL ACETATE: Has been added to perfumes, colognes, shampoos, fabric softeners, stickup air fresheners, dish washing liquids and detergents, soaps, hairs prays, bleaches, aftershaves and deodorants. It is carcinogenic (linked to pancreatic cancer). The vapors are irritating to eyes and respiratory passages, exciting cough. In mice it has caused hyper anemia of the lungs. It can be absorbed through the skin causing systemic effects.*

(This list was compiled by Julia Kendall, Co-Chair , Citizens for a Toxic-Free Marin.)

I could probably cite many additional instances of

the lack of a foolproof system to protect the health of the consumer, therefore, it is wise for the consumer to learn to protect his/her own health. If we are going to be exposed unavoidably to toxins in our food, water, air, cosmetics and medicine, periodic detoxification is a helpful tool to avoid future health complications,

About 70,000 man-made chemicals are being sold today. About 300 have been identified as cancer-causing agents in animal tests by NTP researchers (NIH). "The true number of carcinogenic chemicals is probably far higher, since the program has not conducted even preliminnary screenings on more tha 80 percent of the chemicals currently on the market." Excerpted from *Toxic Deception* p.9.

# Chapter 3
# Symptoms of Toxicity

*When you attack Nature, she comes back again with a pitch-fork* —Dr. Clyde Crumpacker

The body in its wisdom warns us when the systems of elimination are overloaded and there exists a need to detoxify. The body manifests symptoms which are sometimes subtle, but usually become acute enough not to be ignored. If they are understood and handled properly, they can be a beneficial communication to our consciousness to help us maintain our health. The body tries to eliminate toxicity through any of its openings — colon, kidneys, pores, lungs (nose), sometimes through eyes tearing which is rare and ear discharge which is also rare. It discharges toxins via its fluids. The form it takes is not always predictable.

When the normal systems of elimination, colon and kidneys, are overloaded, the body wisely seeks other pathways in its need to get rid of what the immune system considers foreign material. Its first attempt is to sweat the waste out through the pores. If that isn't adequate, it may cause a rash, psoriasis or eczema. Another direction for elimination is through the lungs. This manifests as a runny nose, mucous discharge, coughing and bringing up phlegm. It is sometimes thought to be the flu and unfortunately suppressed with antibiotics before it is determined possibly to be a biological need. If none of these attempts at elimination are sufficient and we do not undertake detoxification, it is then likely that the body will generate a fever or what is sometimes referred to as inflammation. This is Nature's way of taking charge. The fever causes us to go to bed, lose our appetite and drink a lot of liquid. Just what the body requires. As a rule the fever also causes us to sweat profusely thus eliminating toxins naturally through the pores. The act of needing bed rest, taking liquids and sweating allows the body to shift its energy to detoxifying or what I like to call "housecleaning." Mother Nature is a good caretaker. If we pay careful attention and do not violate her instructions, she will attempt to flush out the toxicity. This is actually the work of the immune system maintaining internal cleanliness by eliminating what it considers foreign material.

Fever is not understood well enough in the medical community. It is often a healing process which the body is trying to use efficiently. Whole-body hyperthermia, a system of artificially inducing fever, is used to kill cancer cells. There must be a natural value to fever for it to be able to accomplish tumor reduction by attacking the tumor as foreign material and accomplishing this without harming healthy cells.

Some years ago one of the government agencies, the National Institute of Allergy and Infectious Disease (NIAID), concluded from scientific research that a temperature of up to 104 degrees could be self-limiting.

Boils are another technique the body uses to excrete

toxicity. The late Dr. Bernard Jensen, author of numerous health books and owner and director of a health ranch in Escondido, California, told me he had a patient who had twenty boils at one time. That might represent an unusual need to detoxify, but it also represents an active immune system seeking out foreign material for elimination through any available pathway. *A healthy immune system will not tolerate internal toxicity. It rejects toxicity as it would any foreign material.* If we do not attend to periodic detoxification, and the immune system is healthy, it will attempt to eliminate through any aperture thus causing uncomfortable symptoms. Unfortunately, if the immune system is too weak to effect elimination, the toxic waste will remain stored.

Before taking steps to suppress the body's attempts at "housecleaning" with antibiotics, it might be wiser to wait watchfully to see whether the symptoms need medical attention or are just doing a routine job.

Diarrhea is another pathway the body uses to accommodate waste elimination. It is usually self-limiting, but if it causes weakness or dehydration, steps can be taken to control it.

Edwin Flatto, M.D., in his book about toxicity, *The Restoration of Health Nature's Way*, claims that a headache is "merely the bowels signalling the brain to stop shovelling in fuel until we remove the ashes." The headache, of course, is Nature's way of telling us the body needs relief.

The most subtle indication of toxicity is the loss of our appetite and the desire for liquid. If we take note of the body's communication, the elimination is usually accomplished in a day or two.

     I was listening to a tape of Leo Roy, M.D., a doctor who was exceptionally knowledgeable about the physiology of the body and the importance of avoiding the buildup of toxicity. He was speaking at a convention of the Foundation for Advancement in Cancer Therapy (FACT) about the misuse of vitamins because the unnecessary overload needs to be discarded the same as any waste material. During the question and answer period, a man took the microphone, which was located in the aisle for questioners. He proceeded to disagree with Dr. Roy's statement that vitamins should not be taken indiscriminately without knowing if they were needed. Dr. Roy spoke about his experience with patients who had been using vitamins too casually with disastrous consequences. Typically, the man at the microphone felt his personal experience with vitamins was very beneficial and the universal answer for everyone and possibly every ailment. He wanted the audience to get the benefit of his personal knowledge. Unfortunately, some people in the health movement tend to proselytize when something works for them. They tend to think "one size fits all."

     The man said that he had flu symptoms every year that tended to linger or come back too often until he started taking large doses of vitamin C. Dr. Roy, of course, attempted to make this person understand that the large doses of vitamin C were ***compromising a natural action***. By not allowing the periodic elimination of toxins, he might be building up to a more serious problem than a flu symptom. Unfortunately, it was beyond this man's comprehension.

# Chapter 4

# Detoxification Methods

*Every so-called disease is a crisis of toxemia which means toxins accumulated in the blood above the tolerance point, and the crises are the so-called disease* — J.H.Tilden, M.D.

At natural healing clinics in Europe, Mexico and the United States, the usual procedure is to detoxify a patient before starting a healing program. In this way they control the pace at which the toxicity is released from storage and ready for elimination. The detoxification prepares the body for the repair process which patients are there to accomplish. I am presenting here the detoxification techniques that have been used extensively for many years. There are others but they do not have the same long track record.

## DR. ALAN NITTLER'S DETOXIFICATION

Alan Nittler, M.D., author of the book, *New Breed of Doctor,* had a nutritional practice in California. Before he started his patients on a nutritional program, he detoxified them by putting them on a two-fruit regimen for a period of two weeks. There was no limit to the amount of fruit they could eat. There is always a need to avoid hunger. It is also always important to respond to all vital biological needs.

Of course, Dr. Nittler first decided if the patients were satisfactory candidates for a two-week fruit regimen. For people trying this regimen on one's own, it would be wise to do it for one or two days only, go back to eating for a week or so and then do one or two days again until the symptoms of toxicity have disappeared.

The reason fruits are used to detoxify is because fruits are Natures' cleansers, whereas vegetables are natural body nourishers. The fruit should be of a juicy variety which would not include bananas. This was Dr. Nittler's system before starting a biorepair. It was his way to prepare the body to eliminate its waste before starting a nutritional program to restore host resistance and repair the breakdown in body chemistry. Since the healthier nutritional regimen would break down and replace weaker cells with new cells of bet- ter quality, it was beneficial to remove as much waste as possible at the start of the program. The destroyed cells are a waste product which will be collected by the bloodstream to be processed for elimination. Since these cells are un- healthy, they are treated by the immune system as foreign (toxic) material. While in the bloodstream, they sometimes temporarily cause uncomfortable symptoms, ergo, colon cleansing or a mild herbal laxative is usually recommended to help the body process the elimination efficiently.

## SAUNA

A group of doctors, who have been helping people with chemical sensitivities to detoxify, accomplishes the elimination of stored waste by using a series of saunas. The toxic buildup is eliminated through the pores of the skin through profuse sweating. Some people may be able to accomplish the same results by taking fairly hot Epsom salt baths and then getting under the bed covers to continue sweating as much as possible.

## LIQUID FASTING

A number of clinics in Europe put patients on a liquid fast. This is done under supervision for a period of time determined by the experienced staff. The liquids are available to provide nourishment without using energy for digestion. The body's energy is then diverted to the elimination of toxicity.

The liquids used are tea, usually sweetened with raw honey as the honey contains essential vitamins and minerals, clear vegetable broth, fruit juices and vegetable juices that are diluted with an equal amount of distilled water. Although the person is on a liquid fast, he/she is getting nourishment from the liquids and usually maintains normal energy. The end of the fast is dictated by a feeling of hunger. It is the natural sign that the body needs nourishment so the patient is then returned to a balanced diet.

# GERSON DETOXIFICATION

Dr. Max Gerson ran a clinic in Nanuet, New York where he treated cancer patients as well as patients with many other health problems.. His work is being continued at the Gerson Institute in Tijuana, Mexico. Coffee enemas were used extensively. The infusion was held for at least 12 minutes. The caffein in the coffee stimulated bile flow from the liver which helped the cleansing of the bloodstream. The coffee enemas were given around the clock every four hours or, if indicated, on a three hour schedule. Castor oil, given orally and rectally, was used to clean toxicity from the bowel. This is documented in his book, *A Cancer Therapy, Results of Fifty Cases*. Although this book was written for the medical profession, it has been used by lay people as well. The book is available from FACT, Box 1242 Old Chelsea Station, New York, N. Y. 10113.

## WATER FAST

There are clinics that put patients on a distilled water fast. This is not a do-it-yourself system. It is based on the concept that the body does not have to use its energy for digestion, therefore it shifts its energy to seek out toxins and processes them for elimination. This should be done by experienced practitioners who know who can tolerate a water fast, when to start and when to discontinue it.

## HERBS

28

There are a wide array of herbs that can be used for detoxification. They work in different ways. Some are organ spe-
cific. There are colon cleansers, liver detoxifiers, diuretics,
glandular cleansers, blood cleansers and herbs that cause
sweating. Herbs are usually available at Health Food Stores
with instructions listed on the package.

**Colon**

| | |
|---|---|
| Senna | Cascara segrada |
| Burdock root | Psyllium seeds |

**Liver**

| | |
|---|---|
| Barberry | Burdock root |

**Glandular**

| | |
|---|---|
| Garlic | Capsicum |
| Cayenne pepper | Parsley |

**Kidneys**

| | |
|---|---|
| Barberry | Burdock |
| Yarrow | Parsley |
| Asparagus | Watermelon seeds |

**Blood purifiers**

| | |
|---|---|
| Burdock | Red clover |
| Sarsaparilla | Garlic |
| Turmeric | Burdock |
| Echinacea | Dandelion |

## DR. NORMAN WALKER'S DETOXIFICATION

The most difficult system but most effective for detoxification is one developed by a doctor of science, Norman W. Walker. Not only did he use this for his patients but he used it for himself. Although he lived in a healthy environment and ate healthy food, he routinely did the following detoxification regimen once a year. This was probably responsible for his longevity. He died at the advanced age of 117, quietly in his sleep as normally as one should. He didn't suffer from a long illness as so many people do. Not only that, his mind was clear. His last book was published the year he died. To me he is the best example of a person who knew what he was doing. I consider him one of the outstanding leaders of the health movement. Dr. Walker created the first juice extractor which was named after him. It is the Norwalk juicer and it is still available.

The detoxification method which he created was originally printed in one of the many books he wrote about juicing, diet, stress, pure water and an array of health matters. It is the most aggressive detox system I know of and not necessarily needed for every situation, but there are times when it can correct a very serious case of toxic overload.

Dr. Walker writes in his book, *Raw Vegetable Juices*, "Supreme cleanliness is the first step towards a healthy body. Any accumulation or retention of morbid matter, or waste of any kind, within us, will retard our progress towards recovery."

His detoxification appeared in the book, *Fresh Vegetable Juices*, but was eliminated when it became impossible to get the laxatives suggested in the book as the pharmaceutical company making the laxatives discontinued production as sales were too limited.

Dr. William Donald Kelley, who used Walker's detoxification system for his metabolic program, modified Walker's work for his program by substituting Epsom Salts for the Glauber Salts, Seidlitz Powders or Pluto Water that Walker recommended. This is the way Kelley altered the detoxification:

*Upon arising take one tablespoon of Epsom Salts dissolved in water or juice. In a half hour take the second tablespoon of Epsom Salts dissolved in juice or water. One half hour later take the third dose of Epsom Salts. Then the Walker regimen was continued.*

Prepare a citrus punch made of :

    4 large or 6 medium sized grapefruit

    2 large or 3 medium sized lemons

    And enough oranges to complete a total mixture of Two quarts

    Add to this 2 quarts of distilled water

Dr. Walker writes, "A half hour after taking the saline solution, we drink the citrus punch and continue to drink it for the rest of the day. The purpose of this saline solution is not primarily to empty the bowels, which, however, it will do anyway, but rather to draw into the intestines from every part of the body such toxic matter or body waste as may be present, and to eliminate it through the bowels.

"This saline solution acts on the toxic lymph and body waste just like a magnet acts to attract unto itself nails and metal filings. This body waste is thus drawn into the intestines and out of the body in a series of copious eliminations from the bowel.

"We eat nothing all day, although if hungry, we eat some pieces of fruit or celery juice."

Dr. Walker suggests taking an enema at the end of the day using warm water to clean out the bowel of toxic matter before going to bed. If toxic matter is settled in the colon, it might be absorbed back into the bloodstream during sleep.

"This detoxification is repeated for three consecutive days. On the fourth day, we use a transitional system of eating only raw food for the next three days. On the seventh day, we return to our original diet"

I would suggest if this is undertaken without guidance, to do it for one day only and possibly repeat it for one day weekly until there has been 3 days of detoxification.

Simpler detoxification systems may be more appropriate for a person's lifestyle or need. Perhaps one of those mentioned at the beginning of this chapter would be more suitable for some of our readers.

# Chapter 5
# How to Maintain Health

*Internal cleanliness is more essential than external cleanliness.*

    People often take better care of their cars than of themselves. If the car requires a specific octane of gasoline, that is exactly what the car gets. If it needs the carburetor cleaned (detoxified), it certainly would not be neglected. Why then should we not provide our bodies with the right fuel and keep it as clean as we would any engine?

    Now that we understand the benefits of detoxification and how to do "housecleaning," it might be wise to use our newly acquired knowledge about detoxification to avoid a typical toxic buildup, and in this way avoid some of the health problems that toxicity generates.

    There are foods that provide greater amounts of energy than others and are less likely to produce toxicity. Using these high energy nutrients gives the body its natural ability to detoxify. We also can try to eat foods that are not overloaded with toxic chemicals, i.e., coloring, preservatives, flavor enhancers, stabilizers etc. In this way we lessen the toxic buildup.

    Raw vegetables and fruits have all of the elements that Nature intended for them to be properly digested by humans just as animals have food designed by Nature for them. Raw foods should be part of a wholesome diet in order to acquire the natural elements before they are altered by heat. Nature in its wisdom has done its work competently. All we have to do is cooperate and she will do whatever is necessary. Since the vegetables are the nourishers and fruits the cleansers, we need to provide our bodies with more of the vegetables than the fruit.

Whole grains are a special energy food and should be part of a good balanced regimen. They are a super food for maintaining health. Whole grains contain all the elements needed to produce a new plant and new seeds. That is a special kind of power. And because seeds can reproduce, they automatically have balanced hormones. Balanced hormones might also delay the aging process. Wouldn't it be nice to have our food maintain our health, provide energy and keep us feeling and looking younger instead of using pills or plastic surgery? Some health publications suggest that whole grains will maintain a healthy arterial system.

*"Whole grains are receiving some well-deserved recognition. Research has shown that eating a diet rich in whole grains is associated with significant health benefits, including reduced risk of heart disease, certain types of cancer, and type 2 diabetes, and may also help in weight management."* The above item appeared in the *Food Insight Newsletter*, June 2005, a food trade publication. This newsletter cited all the research from which the information was obtained.

Whole grains provide a wide range of nutrients including good quality organic calcium. These days doctors are urging patients to be aware of osteoporosis. They are urging women to take calcium tablets. Those tablets are usually made of inedible material such as egg shells or sea shells which are difficult or even impossible for the body to metabolize. There is a vast difference in using natural calcium compared to inedible calcium. Natural calcium is absorbed easily by the body and does not risk unmetabolized calcium settling in unpredictable places in the body. Unmetabolized calcium can create serious health problems, i.e., cataracts, arthritis and settlements in the arteries which block circulation and affect the heart. One article, I came across, but could not verify, claimed inedible calcium can cause kidney stones. Whole grains not only contain good quality calcium but contain a wide array of other needed elements, such as, potassium, protein, trace minerals, vitamins B and E and fiber. It's a bonanza!

Add a moderate amount of protein and carbohydrates to your fruits, vegetables, nuts and whole grains and you will have a balanced diet, Some yogurt or any other fermented food will help in the digestive process and maintain balanced intestinal floral. If supplements are used, we need to be sure they are of good quality and right for us. If we are avoiding contaminants in our food, then we certainly don't want them in our supplements.

We can avoid the pollution in our water supply by using distilled water as an excellent substitute. Distillation purifies water by removing all contaminants, chlorine, fluorine, pesticides, inorganic minerals and all residue.

**Avoid** supplements containing coloring, pre-servatives, calcium binders or synthetics.

**Avoid** canola oil. Most oils are made from safe natural products, such as olive oil from olives, peanut oil from peanuts etc. There is *no canola seed* from which to make canola oil. It is made from rapeseed (a poisonous seed that has been genetically engineered (GE) to remove some of the erucic acid, which is a poison. Genetic engineering, unfortunately, does not eliminate the poison entirely! Before the rapeseed was genetically engineered and promoted for human consumption, the oil was used solely for industrial purposes, i.e., to oil machinery.

**Avoid** soy products in large amounts as are suggested by some groups for all our protein, such as soy milk, soy ice cream, soy burgers, soy cheese, soy pudding etc. *Soy is an enzyme inhibitor!* Without enzymatic function, all sorts of health problems can develop. Enzymes are essential for the food we eat to be metabolized (digested) into its microcomponents to be available for the body to use for energy, to repair and, most importantly, for healthy cell production. Undigested food becomes a waste product and adds to the toxic load. The Weston A. Price Foundation, a highly respected nutritional resource, has issued a soy alert!

Following are their conclusions about soy:

* High levels of phytic acid in soy reduces assimilation of calcium, magnesium, copper, iron and zinc. Phytic acid in soy is not neutralized by ordinary preparation methods such as soaking, sprouting and long, slow cooking. High phytate diets have caused growth problems in children.

* Trypsin inhibitors in soy interfere with protein digestion and may cause pancreatic disorders. In test animals soy containing trypsin inhibitors caused stunted growth.

* Soy phytoestrogens disrupt endocrine function and have the potential to cause infertility and promote breast cancer in adult women.

* Soy phytoestrogens are potent antithyroid agents that cause hypothyroidism and may cause thyroid cancer. In infants, consumption of soy formulas has been linked to autoimmune thyroid disease.

* Vitamin B 12 analogs in soy are not absorbed and actually increase the body's requirement for B12.

* Soy foods increase the body's requirement for vitamin D.

* Fragile proteins are denatured during high temperature processing to make soy protein isolate and textured vegetable protein.

* Processing of soy protein results in the formation of toxic lysinoalamine and highly carcinogenic nitrosamines.

* Free glutamic acid or MSG, a potent neurotoxin, is formed during soy food processing and additional amounts are added to many soy foods.

The above list should raise a red flag about the widespread use of soy.

# Chapter 6
# Confusion about Diet and Detoxification

*In healing we have to know that Nature cures, but needs the opportunity to do so. Health depends upon the integrity and activity of every organ in the body. It must be toxic free and chemically balanced.*

*—Dr. Bernard Jensen*

Confusion exists among some practitioners and lay people about the diet and detoxification. They often consider nutrition as a detoxification system. The diet may induce some detoxification but detoxification and diet should be considered as two separate biosystems. The diet is used to restore and repair, whereas, detoxification cleans out the dead cells, unmetabolized food and the toxic chemical buildup from daily living to make the repair process effective. Sometimes, a repair cannot be accomplished until the toxins are eliminated.

Another very serious complication to consider when we start a better nutritional program is the too rapid movement of toxins from storage into the bloodstream and an overloaded colon blocking effective elimination. Starting the flow of toxins, without first clearing a pathway for complete elimination through the colon and kidneys, will cause unpleasant symptoms until the toxins are eliminated from the bloodstream, lymphatics, liver, etc.

If someone is just beginning a change in their dietary intake, as a precaution, it should be done gradually. Too rapid a change can cause the toxic flow to cause an overload of toxins in the bloodstream. This can cause acute discomfort. Headaches, rashes, cough, fever or flu-like symptoms may become evident as the body struggles to eliminate the toxins in the bloodstream. Toxicity develops slowly and needs to be eliminated at a pace the body can handle.

The wisdom of the body will attempt to accomplish the elimination through any of the body's openings until it can effect the relief it is seeking. It uses the pores which may cause a rash; an overload in the bowel may cause diarrhea; the nose may run profusely and sometimes the eyes tear. This is the body's way of relieving the bloodstream. If it is obstructed from reacting normally, ie, through the colon and kidneys, it may temporarily store the toxins in the lymphatic system.

The body will appreciate the cleansing. When the bloodstream is cleared of toxicity, the lymphatics will dump the toxins back into the bloodstream where they can now be processed for complete elimination through the normal channels — the colon and kidney.

Great benefit should be derived from "housecleaning." The body usually responds positively. Nerves are more relaxed. Digestion improves. Energy is revitalized. The mind is clearer. There is a greater zest for life.

# Conclusion

*Health is so necessary to all the duties as well as the plea-*
*sures of life, that the crime of squandering it is equal to the folly.*
— *Dr. Samuel Johnson*

Now that we know the hazards of toxicity and the benefits
of detoxification, it would be foolhardy to waste the advantages of
periodically detoxifying and enjoying the benefits which are im-
measurable.

Not only can we avoid future health problems from a toxic
buildup but, the mind is clearer so we make more logical decisions.
We find ourselves more relaxed and able to cope with problems in
spite of hectic times or nerve-wracking conditions. The nervous
system which is usually irritated by the toxins, which are acidic and
sap our strength, are relieved of the toxic irritating burden.

It is my hope that writing this book was worthwhile and that
it will contribute to the health and happiness of the reader.

# About The Author:

*ounder, Foundation for Advancement in Cancer Therapy (F.A.C.T.)*
uth Sackman served as President and Co-Founder of F.A.C.T. for
7 years until her death in December 2008. As a young woman,
ne began as a seamstress and ultimately achieved success as a
esigner. With this success, she dedicated herself to raising her
nildren and became active in her community.

uth's life abruptly changed when her daughter Arlene was diag-
osed with acute leukemia. Despite Ruth's fulltime dedication,
rlene died a year later, after undergoing traditional chemotherapy.
he loss set Ruth on her lifelong quest to find another, better way to
eat cancer.

1971, Ruth and her husband Leon co-founded F.A.C.T. from their
ome in New York. Being head of F.A.C.T. gave Ruth the opportu-
ty to hear from literally thousands of cancer patients worldwide
ver the years, as they experienced the multitude of treatments
vailable in both the conventional as well as non-conventional can-
er areas. This gave her a vast understanding of these many thera-
ies.

uth also personally investigated and consulted with hundreds of
ractitioners and medical clinics around the globe. She hosted a
all-in health program on nationally-syndicated radio, as well as
eing a frequent guest on radio and TV shows nationwide, and was
ditor-in-chief of *Cancer Forum*, F.A.C.T.'s quarterly magazine.

uth authored two books that present F.A.C.T.'s guiding principles
nd the case studies of patients who followed F.A.C.T.'s protocol
nd have rid themselves of disease. This is the core inspiration for
ie documentary, *Rethinking Cancer*. For more information please
sit www.rethinkingcancer.org.